C000131793

Table of Contents

MATH REQUIREMENTS

One of the major objectives of nursing is that the student be able to administer medications safely. In order to meet this objective, the student must be able to meet the following math competencies.

1. Translate Arabic numbers to Roman numerals.
2. Translate Roman numerals to Arabic numbers.
3. Add, subtract, multiply and divide whole numbers.
4. Add, subtract, multiply and divide fractions.
5. Add, subtract, multiply and divide decimals.
6. Convert decimals to percents.
7. Convert percents to decimals.
8. Set up and solve ratio and proportion problems.
9. Convert from one system of measure to another using:
   a) metric system
   b) apothecary system
   c) household system
10. Solve drug problems involving non-parenteral and parental medications utilizing metric, apothecary, and household systems of measurement.
11. Solve IV drip rate problems.

Preparation for the math in nursing is a personal independent student activity. In order to facilitate this task it is suggested that the student utilize an organized approach.

1. Take the self-diagnostic math test. Allow 1 hour for self-test.
2. Use an assessment sheet to pinpoint problem areas.
3. Use the suggested resources to work on the problem areas.
4. Retake the diagnostic test to determine the need for further help.

Students are encouraged to follow the above procedures. It will organize their own learning efforts and also serve as a basis for assistance from tutors or clinical instructors.

*NOTE: **Part G – IV Drip Calculations** contains material that will be tested on after the first semester. Refer to this section beginning in the second semester to solve practice problems.

MATH LEARNING RESOURCES

1.   This booklet, <u>Fundamentals of Mathematics for Nursing</u>.

2.   Self-diagnostic math tests - enclosed.

3.   General math text - Sixth grade math books will include material on whole numbers, fractions, decimals, and ratio and proportion.

      Middle School math books will include material on solving for an unknown.

      These texts can be obtained from school or public libraries.

4.   College of Health Sciences -- Learning Resource Center (LRC) -- Rowlett 310 -- 622-3576

      Math text -- <u>NURSING MATH SIMPLIFIED</u> -- available in LRC.

5.   <u>The following computer programs are available in the LRC.:</u>

      <u>CALCULATE WITH CARE</u>

      Comprehensive self-study computer program. Where users learn independently at their own pace . . . take notes, write down a rule, do practice problems, get immediate feedback on the answers, review as often as necessary. The program uses realistic problems and provides all the information needed to solve them.

      <u>MED PREP</u>

      <u>DOSAGES & SOLUTIONS</u>

      <u>IM MEDS</u>

Conversions

There are three measurement systems commonly used in health care facilities: the metric, household, and apothecary system. In order to compare measured amounts in the systems, <u>approximate equivalents</u> have been developed. An example of an approximate equivalent is 1 teaspoon is approximately equal to 5 milliliters. Because the measures are <u>not exactly equal</u>, a conversion which takes more than one step will not produce as accurate a value as a conversion which takes only one step. For example, it is more accurate to convert from teaspoon to milliliters by using the conversion factor directly from teaspoons to milliliters than it is to go from teaspoons to ounces to milliliters.

<u>RULE</u>: Always convert from one unit of measure to another by the shortest number of steps possible.

Systems of Measurement and Approximate Equivalents

The following conversion table will have to be memorized in order to accurately calculate dosage problems.

Metric	Apothecaries	Household
VOLUME		
	1 minim (m)	1 drop (gtt)
1 milliliter (ml)(cc)	15-16 minims (m)	15-16 gtts
4 milliliters (ml) (cc)	1 dram (dr), (4 ml's or cc's)	1 teaspoon (t) (4-5 cc), 60 drops (gtts)
15 milliliters (ml) (cc)		1 tablespoon (T), 3 teaspoons (t)
30 milliliters (ml) (cc)	1 ounce (oz)	2 tablespoon (T)
1000 milliliter (1 liter)	1 quart	1 quart

WEIGHT		
1 milligram (mg)	1000 micrograms (mcg)	
60 milligrams (mg)	1 grain (gr)	
1 gram (gm)	15 grains (gr), 1000 milligrams (mg)	
454 grams (gm)	16 ounces (oz)	1 pound (lb)
1 Kilogram (Kg)		2.2 pounds (lb)

Units (u) and milliequivalents (meq) **cannot** be converted to units in other systems. They have their value given and will never need to be converted.
1 unit – 1000 miliunits
*Cubic centimeters (cc's) and milliliters (ml's) can be used interchangeably.

Common Pharmacologic Abbreviations

To transcribe medication orders and document drug administration accurately, review the following commonly used abbreviations for drug measurements, dosage forms, routes and times of administration, and related terms. Remember that abbreviations often are subject to misinterpretation especially if written carelessly or quickly. If an abbreviation seems unusual or doesn't make sense to you, given your knowledge of the patient or the drug, always question the order, clarify the terms, and clearly write out the correct term in your revision and transcription.

DRUG AND SOLUTION MEASUREMENTS

cc	cubic centimeter
D, dr	dram
oz.	Ounce
G, gm	gram
gr	grain
gtt	drop
Kg	kilogram
L	liter
mcg	microgram
mEq	milliequivalent
mg	milligram
ml	milliliter
m	minim
pt	pint
qt	quart
ss	one-half
Tbs, T	tablespoon
Tsp, t	teaspoon
U	unit
mu	milliunit

DRUG DOSAGE FORMS

cap	capsule
DS	double strength
EC	enteric coated
Elix	elixir
Liq	liquid
Sol	solution
Supp	suppository
Susp	suspension
Syr	syrup
Tab	tablet
Ung, oit	ointment

ROUTES OF DRUG ADMINISTRATION

AS	left ear
AD	right ear
AU	each ear
IM	intramuscular
IV	intravenous
IVPB	intravenous piggyback
V, PV	vaginally
OS	left eye
OD	right eye
OU	each eye
PO	by mouth
R, PR	by rectum
R	right
L	left
SC, SQ	subcutaneous
S&S	swish & swallow

TIMES OF DRUG ADMINISTRATION

ac	before meals
ad lib	as desired
Bid	twice a day
HS	at bedtime
pc	after meals
Prn	as needed
Q am, QM	every morning
QD, qd	every day
Qh	every hour
Q2h	every 2 hours
Q3h	every 3 hours, and so on
Qid	four times a day
Qod	every other day
STAT	immediately
Tid	three times a day

COMMON INTRAVENOUS FLUIDS

D_5W – 5% Dextrose in water
D_5NS – 5% Dextrose in normal saline
D_5 ½NS – 5% Dexrose in ½ normal saline
L.R. – Lactated Ringers
Remember 1 liter = 1000 ml

MISCELLANEOUS

AMA	against medical advise
ASA	aspirin
ASAP	as soon as possible
BS	blood sugar (glucose)
c	with
C/O	complains of
D/C	discontinue
DX	diagnosis
HX	history
KVO	keep vein open
MR	may repeat
NKA	no known allergies
NKDA	no known drug allergies
NPO	nothing by mouth
R/O	rule out
R/T	related to
Rx	treatment, prescription
s	without
S/S	signs/symptoms
Sx	symptoms
TO	telephone order
VO	verbal order
~	approximately equal to
>	greater than
<	less than
↑	increase
↓	decrease

PART A
BASIC MATH REVIEW

The following section serves as a review of basic math principles and allows students to identify any areas that will require further study. Students who find they need further development in basic math should refer to the table of math resources on page 5. Answers for practice problems are located in Part G, beginning on page 48.

1.	Roman Numerals

$I = 1$ $V = 5$ $X = 10$ $L = 50$ $C = 100$ $D = 500$ $M = 1000$

The basic form is to place the <u>larger numerals to the left</u> and add other numerals.

   XXXIII = 33   (30 + 3 = 33)

There is an exception to the basic form.
If <u>smaller numeral precedes a larger numeral</u>, the smaller should be subtracted from the larger.

   IX = 9   (1 - 10 = 9)

If there seems to be several ways of writing a number - use the shorter form.

   XVVI - incorrect
   XXI - correct
   (10 + 10 + 1 = 21)

<u>Only one smaller numeral</u> is allowed to precede a larger numeral.

   XCV = 95 - correct
   IXCV - incorrect
   (10 - 100 = 90 + 5 = 95)

Numerals may be written as <u>lower case letters</u> and the <u>number one</u> may have a line and/or a dot over it.

   iv = 4 $\dot{\bar{1}} = 1$ $xv\ddot{1}1 = 17$
   1 - 5 = 4   10 + 5 + 2 = 17

2. Fractions

Numerator
Denominator

$\frac{2}{3}$ = Proper fraction = numerator is <u>smaller</u> than denominator.

$\frac{3}{2}$ = Improper faction = numerator is <u>larger</u> than denominator.

$1\frac{1}{2}$ = Mixed fraction = whole number and a fraction.

To change an improper fraction to a mixed number:
a. Divide the numerator by the denominator. $\frac{13}{5} = 2\frac{3}{5}$
b. Place remainder over denominator.

To change a mixed number to an improper fraction:
a. Multiply denominator by the whole number. $3\frac{1}{2} = \frac{7}{2}$
b. Add numerator.
c. Place sum over the denominator.

To reduce a fraction to its lowest denominator:
a. Divide numerator and denominator by the greatest common divisor.
b. The value of the fraction does not change.

   EXAMPLE: Reduce $\frac{12}{60}$

      12 divides evenly into both numerator and denominator

      $12 \div 12 = 1$ $\frac{12}{60} = \frac{1}{5}$
      $60 \div 12 = 5$

   EXAMPLE: Reduce $\frac{9}{12}$

      3 divides evenly into both

      $9 \div 3 = 3$
      $12 \div 3 = 4$

      $\frac{9}{12} = \frac{3}{4}$

EXAMPLE: Reduce $\dfrac{30}{45}$

15 divides evenly into both

$30 \div 15 = 2$
$45 \div 15 = 3$

$\dfrac{30}{45} = \dfrac{2}{3}$

You can multiply or divide when denominators are <u>NOT</u> alike. You <u>CANNOT</u> add or subtract unless the fractions have the same denominator.

Addition of fractions:
a. Must have common denominator.
b. Add numerators.

$\dfrac{1}{4} + \dfrac{2}{8} = \left(\text{change } \dfrac{2}{8} \text{ to } \dfrac{1}{4}\right) = \dfrac{1}{4} + \dfrac{1}{4} = \dfrac{2}{4} = \dfrac{1}{2}$

Subtraction of fractions:
a. Must have common denominator.
b. Subtract numerators.

$\dfrac{6}{8} - \dfrac{3}{4} = \left(\text{change } \dfrac{6}{8} \text{ to } \dfrac{3}{4}\right) = \dfrac{3}{4} - \dfrac{3}{4} = 0$

Multiplication of fractions:
a.   To multiply a fraction by a whole number, multiply numerator by the whole number and place product over denominator.

$4 \times \dfrac{3}{8} = \dfrac{12}{8} = 1\dfrac{4}{8} = 1\dfrac{1}{2}$

b.   To multiply a fraction by another fraction, multiply numerators and denominators.

$\dfrac{5}{6} \times \dfrac{3}{4} = \dfrac{15}{24} = \dfrac{5}{8}$

Division of fractions:
a. Invert terms of divisor.
b. Then multiply.

EXAMPLE 1: $\dfrac{2}{3} \div \dfrac{4}{5}$

$\dfrac{2}{3} \times \dfrac{5}{4} = \dfrac{10}{12}$ Reduced to lowest terms $= \dfrac{5}{6}$

EXAMPLE 2: $4 \div \dfrac{5}{6}$

$$4 \times \dfrac{6}{5} = \dfrac{24}{5} = 4\dfrac{4}{5}$$

3. Decimals

millions	hundred thousands	ten thousands (10,000)	thousands (1000)	hundreds (100)	tens (1)	ones (1)	tenths (0.1)	hundredths (0.01)	thousandths (0.001)	ten thousandths	hundred thousandths	millionths

_____Decimal _____
To the left   Point   To the right

Reading from right to left, each place is 10 times larger in value. For example, 100 is 10 times larger than 10 and 1.0 is 10 times larger than 0.1.

Changing decimals to fractions:

a.   Express the decimal in words.
b.   Write the words as a fraction
c.   Reduce to lowest terms.

EXAMPLE 1:   0.3

a. three tenths   b. $\dfrac{3}{10}$ c. already reduced to lowest terms

EXAMPLE 2: 0.84

a. eighty-four hundredths   b. $\dfrac{84}{100}$ c. $\dfrac{21}{25}$

Changing fractions to decimals:

Divide the numerator by the denominator.

EXAMPLE 1: $\dfrac{3}{4}$ 4 $\overline{\smash{\big)}\,3.00}$ $\dfrac{.75}{}$ so $\dfrac{3}{4}$ = 0.75
                    28
                    20
                    20
                     0

EXAMPLE 2: $\dfrac{8}{40}$ 40 $\overline{\smash{\big)}\,8.0}$ $\dfrac{.2}{}$ so $\dfrac{8}{40}$ = 0.2
                    80
                     0

Addition and Subtraction of decimals:

Use the decimal point as a guide and line up the numbers by their decimal place so that all the ones places are lined up under each other, all the tens places lined up and so on.

ADDITION EXAMPLE 1:   7.4
                    +12.39
                     19.79

ADDITION EXAMPLE 2:   .003
                       2.4
                       .15
                    + .02157
                     2.57457

SUBTRACTION EXAMPLE 1: 86.4
                     - 3.817
                      82.583

SUBTRACTION EXAMPLE 2: 6.079
                      - .85
                       5.229

Multiplication of decimals:

a. Multiply the numbers as if they were whole numbers.
b. Count the total number of decimal places to the right of the decimal point for each
        of the numbers.
c. Use that total to count decimal places in the answer.

a. 17.3   17.3
   x 0.45 x 0.45
            865
            692
        7785 = 7.785

b. 17.3 has 1 decimal place past the decimal point.

   .45 has 2 decimal places past the decimal point
            3 total

c. Count 3 places for decimal in answer - 7.785

Division of decimals:

To divide a decimal by a whole number, the decimal is placed directly above the decimal in the dividend.

```
     Quotient                1.37
Divisor | Dividend       5 | 6.85
                              5
                             ──
                             18
                             15
                             ──
                             35
                             35
                             ──
                              0
```

To divide a decimal by a decimal:

Shift the decimal of the divisor enough places to make it a whole number. The decimal in the dividend is moved the same number of places as the divisor. Decimal point of quotient is placed directly above the new place of the decimal in the dividend.

```
                        .                5.
EXAMPLE 1:   .6 | 3.0         6 | 30.0
                                   30
                                   ──
                                    0
```

```
                        .               17.2
EXAMPLE 2:   1.3 | 22.36      13 | 223.6
                                   13
                                   ──
                                   93
                                   91
                                   ──
                                   26
                                   26
                                   ──
```

Rounding off decimals:

Decide how far the number is to be rounded, such as to the tenths place or the hundredths place. Mark that place by putting a line under it.

If the digit to the right of that place is less than 5, drop that digit and any others to the right. If the digit to the right of the place to be rounded to is 5 or greater, increase the number in the place by 1 and drop the digits to the right.

EXAMPLE 1: 7.4 2 3957   7.42

Rounded to nearest hundredth

EXAMPLE 2: 87.852   87.9

Rounded to nearest tenth

Rules for rounding off for nursing math tests:

1. At the end of each step round the answer to the nearest hundredths before proceeding to the next step.
2. If the final answer is less than one, the answer should be rounded off to hundredths, Example .6666   .67
3. If the final answer is greater than one, the answer should be rounded to tenths, Example 1.812   1.8
4. In IV problems, round to the nearest whole number. Therefore, you must round the final answer up if equal to or greater than .5 and round down if less than .5. See example, page 46. If the question states that the IV solution is administered by IV pump, the final answer must be rounded to the nearest hundredth.

4. Practice Problems

Basic Math Practice
Practice #1
Roman Numerals

1. xvi = _____

2. CDXII = _____

3. XLVII = _____

4. XXi =

5. XLIV =

6. MCXX =

7. 54 =

8. 29 =

9. 83 =

10. $2\frac{1}{2}$ = _____

ANSWERS: Page 60

Practice #2
Fractions

1. $\frac{15}{2}$ =

2. $\frac{13}{6}$ =

3. $\frac{7}{4}$ =

4. $\frac{11}{3}$ =

5. $\frac{15}{8}$ =

6. $\frac{37}{5}$ =

7. $\dfrac{4}{6} =$

8. $\dfrac{3}{9} =$

9. $\dfrac{15}{60} =$

10. $\dfrac{1}{16} + \dfrac{4}{5} + \dfrac{3}{4} =$

11. $\dfrac{5}{9} + \dfrac{2}{5} =$

12. $\dfrac{2}{7} + \dfrac{1}{2} + \dfrac{9}{14} =$

13. $\dfrac{1}{2} - \dfrac{1}{3} =$

14. $\dfrac{9}{12} - \dfrac{3}{4} =$

15. $\dfrac{6}{7} - \dfrac{2}{3} =$

16. $\dfrac{7}{8} \times \dfrac{2}{3} =$

17. $1\dfrac{1}{2} \times \dfrac{3}{4} =$

18. $\dfrac{12}{25} \times \dfrac{1}{100} =$

19. $\dfrac{2}{8} \div \dfrac{1}{2} =$

20. $1\dfrac{2}{3} \div \dfrac{1}{3} =$

21. $2\dfrac{1}{2} \div \dfrac{1}{6} =$

22. $\dfrac{2}{9} \div \dfrac{1}{2} =$

ANSWERS: Page 60

Practice # 3
Decimals

Change fractions to decimals

1. $\frac{6}{8}$ =

2. $\frac{5}{10}$ =

3. $\frac{3}{8}$ =

4. $\frac{2}{3}$ =

Change decimals to fractions

5. 0.54 =

6. 0.154 =

7. 0.60 =

8. 0.2 =

Add decimals

9. 1.64 + 0.6 =

10. 0.02 + 1.0 =

11. 2.63 + .01 =

12. 1.54 + 0.3 =

Subtract decimals

13. 1.23 - 0.6 =

14. 0.02 - 0.01 =

15. 2.45 - 0.03 =

16. 0.45 - 0.02 =

Multiply decimals

17. 0.23 x 1.63 =

18. .03 x 0.123 =

19. 1.45 x 1.63 =

20. 0.2 x 0.03 =

Divide

21. 3.2 ÷ 4 =

22. 1.86 ÷ 3.0 =

23. 1.00 ÷ 25 =

24. 68.8 ÷ 2.15 =

Round to hundredths

25. 0.4537 =

26. 0.00584 =

Round to tenths

27. 9.888 =

28. 50.09186 =

Round to tens

29. 5619.94 =

30. 79.13 =

ANSWERS: Page 61

PART B
MEASUREMENT SYSTEMS

1. Ratios and Proportions

The faculty is aware that ratio/proportional problems can be set up in several forms to solve the problem. We believe the fractional form is more conceptual in nature. The fractional form helps the student visualize what is ordered and is available to determine the correct amount of medication to administer.

Students will be required to set up all dosage calculation problems in the fractional form. This method is demonstrated on the following pages:

A ratio compares 2 quantities and can be written as a fraction, 3 to 4 or $\frac{3}{4}$.

4 quarters to 1 dollar is a ratio and can be written $\frac{4}{1}$ or 4:1.

(Other familiar ratios are 60 minutes to 1 hour; 2 cups to 1 pint; 16 ounces to 1 pound).

A proportion is 2 ratios equal to each other.

$$\frac{4 \text{ quarters}}{1 \text{ dollar}} = \frac{8 \text{ quarters}}{2 \text{ dollars}}$$

This proportion can be read 4 quarters are to 1 dollar as 8 quarters are to 2 dollars.

In a proportion, the products of cross multiplication are equal. Using the proportion above:

$$\frac{4}{1} = \frac{8}{2} \qquad 4(2) = 1(8) \qquad 8 = 8$$

There are 4 basic steps to solving proportion problems:

1) Set up a known ratio.
2) Set up a proportion with known and desired units. Use x for the quantity that is desired or unknown.

Be sure the units are the same horizontally.

EXAMPLE: $\dfrac{\text{ounces}}{\text{pounds}} = \dfrac{\text{ounces}}{\text{pounds}}$

3) Cross multiply.
4) Solve for x.

To solve a proportion problem such as 3 lbs. = ? ounces:

a) Set up a known ratio of pounds to ounces.

   1 lb.: 16 oz.

b) Make a proportion using the known ratio on one side and the desired ratio on the other.

   $$\frac{16 \text{ oz.}}{1 \text{ lb.}} = \frac{x \text{ oz.}}{3 \text{ lbs.}}$$

   Be sure the units are the same horizontally, such as ounces on the top and pounds on the bottom of each ratio.

c) Cross multiply.

$$\frac{16 \text{ oz.}}{1 \text{ lb.}} = \frac{x \text{ oz.}}{3 \text{ lbs.}} \qquad 16(3) = 1(x)$$

d) Solve for x.

$$1(x) = 16(3)$$

$$X = 48$$

Therefore, 3 lbs. = 48 ounces.

Another name for a ratio with numerator and denominator of approximately the same value is a <u>conversion factor</u>. The ratios 4 quarters to 1 dollar and 2 pints to 1 quart are conversion factors. Systems of measure use conversion factors to change from one unit to another.

2. Metric System

The basic unit of weight in the metric system is the gram (G or gm.). The basic length is the meter (m) and the basic volume is the liter (l or L). Metric measurements uses the decimal system as the basis for its units. The prefix of the unit identifies its decimal location and value.

micro (mc) = millionths milli (m) – thousandths centi (c)= hundredths deci (d) = tenths deka (da) = tens hecto (h) = hundreds Kilo (k) = thousands	thousands = KILO	hundreds = HECTO	tens = DEKA	ones = Basic Unit	tenths = DECI	hundredths = CENTI	thousandths = MILLI	millionths = MICRO
	larger			Decimal Point	smaller			

The faculty desire that you use a ratio and proportion format to make conversions within the metric system.

Conversion Examples

1. 0.5 G = _____ mg. $\dfrac{1000 \text{ mg}}{1 \text{ G}} = \dfrac{x \text{ mg}}{0.5 \text{ G}}$

    $1(x) = 1000 (0.5)$

    $x = 500 \text{ mg}$

2. 2000 mcg = _____ mg. $\dfrac{1000 \text{ mcg}}{1 \text{ mg}} = \dfrac{2000 \text{ mcg}}{x \text{ mg}}$

    $1000(x) = 2000 (1)$

    $1000x = 2000$

    $x = 2 \text{ mg}$

3.   Practice Problems

METRIC SYSTEM PRACTICE #4 PROBLEMS

1. 7 kg = _____ gm   2. 0.05 l = _____ ml

3. 2.5 gm = _____ mg   4. 5.07 kg = _____ gm

5.	0.5 ml = _____ 1	6.	.0193 1 = _____ ml

7.	1.34 kg = _____ mg	8.	3.7 mg = _____ gm

ANSWERS: Page 62

4.	Household System

This system of measure is not as accurate as the metric or apothecary systems.

The units of volume include drop (gtts), teaspoon (tsp or t.), tablespoon (tbsp. or T) and ounces (oz.).

1 tsp = 60 gtts
1 tbsp. = 3 tsp.
1 oz. = 2 tbsp.

Conversion example:	4 tsp. = X gtts

$$\frac{60 \text{ gtts}}{1 \text{ tsp.}} = \frac{x \text{ gtt}}{4 \text{ tsp.}}$$

60(4) = 1(x)

240 = x

4 tsp. = 240 gtts

5.	Practice Problems

HOUSEHOLD CONVERSION PRACTICE #5 PROBLEMS

1.	2 tsp. = _____ gtt	2.	1 $\underline{1}$ tbsp. = _____ tsp.
				2

3.	45 gtts = _____ tsp.	4.	5 tbsp. = _____ oz.

5.	8 oz. = _____ tbsp.	6.	12 tsp. = _____ tbsp.

ANSWERS: Page 62

PART C
DOSAGE CALCULATIONS

1.   Single-Step Calculation

Medication may be ordered in a form or amount different from what is available.
Proportion may be used to calculate the right dosage.

Steps:

a.   Set up proportion.
b.   Check to be sure units are the same horizontally.
c.   Cross multiply and solve for x.

EXAMPLE 1:

60 mg of medication are ordered. Tablets are available which have 30 mg of
medication in each of them. How many tablets are needed to give 60 mg?

a)   Set up the problem as a proportion. 30 mg are to 1 tablet as 60 mg are to X
tablets.

$$\frac{30 \text{ mg}}{1 \text{ tab}} = \frac{60 \text{ mg}}{x \text{ tab}}$$

b)   Remember to have the same units horizontally (mg to mg and tablets to tablets).

c)   Cross multiply and solve for x.

$$30x = 60$$

$$x = \frac{60}{30} = 2$$

2 tablets = 60 mg = the amount of medication ordered

EXAMPLE 2:

Ordered: 15 mEq
Available: 10 mEq/5cc
How many cc's needed?

a)   Set up proportion.

$$\frac{10 \text{ mEq}}{5 \text{ cc}} = \frac{15 \text{ mEq}}{x \text{ cc}}$$

b) Units are matched therefore no need to convert (mEq to mEq and cc to cc)

c) Cross multiply and solve for x.

$$10x = 75 \quad x = \frac{75}{10} = 7.5 \quad\quad 15 \text{ mEq} = 7.5 \text{ cc}$$

EXAMPLE 3:

Ordered: gr $\frac{1}{800}$

Available: gr $\frac{1}{200}$ per ml

How many mls?

a) Set up proportion.

$$\frac{\frac{1}{200} \text{ gr}}{1 \text{ ml}} = \frac{\frac{1}{800} \text{ gr}}{\text{x ml}}$$

b) Units are the same horizontally.

c) Cross multiply and solve for x.

$$\frac{1}{200}(x) = \frac{1}{800}(1)$$

$$x = \frac{\frac{1}{800}}{\frac{1}{200}} = \frac{1}{800} \text{ X } \frac{200}{1}$$

$$x = \frac{200}{800} = \frac{1}{4} = .25$$

gr $\frac{1}{800}$ = .25 ml

2.	Multiple-Step Calculations

It may be necessary to convert from one unit to another first before solving a dosage problem.

Steps:

a)   Set up proportion.

b)   Convert to like units.

c)   Substitute converted unit into the proportion.

d)   Cross multiply and solve for x.

EXAMPLE 1:

240 mg are ordered. Medication is available in 2 grains/1 tablet. How many tablets should be given?

a) Set up proportion.

$\dfrac{2\ gr}{1\ tab} = \dfrac{240\ mg}{x\ tab}$ Units do not match.

b) Convert to like units.

The units are not alike so grains need to be converted to milligrams or milligrams to grains. It is usually more convenient to convert to the units of the tablet or liquid. Therefore in this problem convert milligrams to grains.

1 gr = 60 mg

$\dfrac{1\ gr}{60\ mg} = \dfrac{x\ gr}{240\ mg}$

240 = 60x

$\dfrac{240}{60} = x$

4 = x

x = 4 gr

c) Now substitute in the original proportion so the units now match.

$\dfrac{2\ gr}{1\ tab} = \dfrac{4\ gr}{x\ tab}$

d) Cross multiply and solve for x.

$2x = 4(1)$

$x = \dfrac{4}{2} = 2$

$x = 2$ tablets

EXAMPLE 2:

Ordered: 0.016 gm

Available: 4 mg/1 ml

How many ml should be given?

a) Set up proportion.

$\dfrac{4 \text{ mg}}{1 \text{ ml}} = \dfrac{0.016 \text{ gm}}{x \text{ ml}}$ Units do not match.

b) Convert to like units.

$\dfrac{1 \text{ gm}}{1000 \text{ mg}} = \dfrac{0.016 \text{ gm}}{x \text{ mg}}$ $x = 1000\,(0.016)$
$x = 16$ mg

c) Substitute converted units into proportion.

$\dfrac{4 \text{ mg}}{1 \text{ ml}} = \dfrac{16 \text{ mg}}{x \text{ ml}}$

d) Cross multiply and solve for x.

$4x = 1(16)$

$x = \dfrac{16}{4} = 4$

$x = 4$ ml

EXAMPLE 3:

Ordered: gr x̄ss orally
Available: 0.3 gm/5 cc

How many cc's should be given?

a) Set up proportion

$$\frac{0.3 \text{ gm}}{5 \text{ cc}} = \frac{\text{gr xss}}{\text{x cc}} \qquad \text{ss} = .5 \text{ or } \frac{1}{2}$$

b) Convert to like units (grains or grams or grams to grains)

$$\frac{15 \text{ gr}}{1 \text{ gm}} = \frac{10.5 \text{ gr}}{\text{x gm}}$$

$$15x = 10.5$$

$$x = 0.7 \text{ gm}$$

c) Substitute converted units into the proportion.

$$\frac{0.3 \text{ gm}}{5 \text{ cc}} = \frac{0.7 \text{ gm}}{\text{x cc}}$$

d) Cross multiply and solve for x.

$$0.3x = 3.5$$

$$x = \frac{3.5}{0.3} = 11.7$$

$$x = 11.7 \text{ cc's}$$

EXAMPLE 4:

Ordered: Two tablespoons of a liquid every 2 hours for 12 hours. How many cc's of the drug will the client receive over the 12 hour period?

a) Set up proportion. $\frac{2 \text{ Tbsp}}{2 \text{ hours}} = \frac{\text{xcc}}{12 \text{ hrs.}}$

b) Convert to like units. $\frac{15 \text{ cc}}{1 \text{ Tbsp.}} = \frac{\text{xcc}}{2 \text{ Tbsp.}}$ $1x = 30$ $x = 30$

c) Substitute converted units into the proportion.

$$\frac{30 \text{ cc}}{2 \text{ hours}} = \frac{\text{xcc}}{12 \text{ hours}}$$

d) Cross multiply and solve for x.

$$\frac{30 \text{ cc}}{2 \text{ hours}} = \frac{\text{xcc}}{12 \text{ hours}} \qquad \begin{array}{l} 2x = 360 \\ x = 180 \text{ cc} \end{array}$$

The client will receive 180cc over a 12 hour period.

EXAMPLE 5:

A client is to receive 2 gm of a drug. The drug comes 500 mg/5 cc. Each vial contains 10 cc's. How many vials would you need?

$$\frac{2 \text{ gm}}{\text{xcc}} = \frac{500 \text{ mg}}{5 \text{ cc}}$$

1. $\dfrac{2 \text{ gm}}{\text{x mg}} = \dfrac{1 \text{ gm}}{1000 \text{ mg}}$

 2. $\dfrac{500 \text{ mg}}{5 \text{ cc}} = \dfrac{2000 \text{ mg}}{\text{xcc}}$

 $1x = 1000(2)$

 $500x = (5) \, 2000$

 $\dfrac{1x}{1} = \dfrac{2000}{1}$

 $\dfrac{500x}{500} = \dfrac{10,000}{500}$

 $x = 2000 \text{ mg}$

 $x = 20 \text{ cc}$

3. $\dfrac{10 \text{ cc}}{1 \text{ vial}} = \dfrac{20 \text{ cc}}{\text{x vial}}$

 $10x = (1) \, 20$

 $\dfrac{10x}{10} = \dfrac{20}{10}$

 $x = 2 \text{ vials}$

3.	Dosage by Weight

Order: 25 mg/kg of body wt.
Available: 5 gm/20 cc
How many cc's do you give to a 30 lb. child?

The order first needs to be clarified to establish exactly what has been ordered.

STEP 1:

1.   Clarify the order (How much medicine is 25 mg/kg for a 30 lb. patient?)

a)   Set up proportion.

 $\dfrac{25 \text{ mg}}{1 \text{ kg}} = \dfrac{\text{x mg}}{30 \text{ lbs}}$ Units don't match so they must be converted.

b)   Convert to like units.

$$\frac{2.2 \text{ lbs.}}{1 \text{ kg}} = \frac{30 \text{ lbs.}}{x \text{ kg}}$$

$2.2x = 30$

$$x = \frac{30}{2.2} = 13.64 \text{ kg}$$

(NOTE: Remember to round the Kg to hundredths place before continuing with the problem)

c) Substitute converted units into the original proportion.

$$\frac{25 \text{ mg}}{1 \text{ kg}} = \frac{x \text{ mg}}{13.64 \text{ kg}}$$

$(1)x = 25(13.64)$

$x = 341 \text{ mg}$

STEP 2:

Now, as in previous problems a proportion is set up with what is ordered and what medicine is on hand (available).

a) Set up proportion.

$$\frac{5 \text{ gm}}{20 \text{ cc}} = \frac{341 \text{ mg}}{x \text{ cc}}$$

b) Convert to like units.

$$\frac{1 \text{ gm}}{1000 \text{ mg}} = \frac{x \text{ gm}}{341 \text{ mg}}$$

$1000x = 341$

$x = 0.341 \text{ gm}$　　　$x = 0.34 \text{ gm}$

c) Substitute converted units and solve for x.

$$\frac{5 \text{ gm}}{20 \text{ cc}} = \frac{0.34 \text{ gm}}{x \text{ cc}}$$

$5x = 20 (0.34)$

$5x = 6.8$

$x = \dfrac{6.8}{5} = 1.364 \text{ cc}$ (final answer rounded to 1.4 cc per rounding rules)

Give 1.4 cc to 30 lb child ordered to have 25 mg/kg of body wt.

A twenty-two pound infant is to receive 2 mg/kg of a drug. The drug is available in 10 mg/.5 cc. How many cc's will be given?

$$\frac{22 \text{ lbs}}{x \text{ mg}} = \frac{1 \text{ kg}}{2 \text{ mg}}$$

1. $$\frac{22 \text{ lbs}}{x \text{ kg}} = \frac{2.2 \text{ lbs}}{1 \text{ kg}}$$

   $$\frac{2.2x}{2.2} = \frac{(1) \ 22}{2.2}$$

   $$x = 10 \text{ kg}$$

2. $$\frac{2 \text{ mg}}{1 \text{ kg}} = \frac{x \text{ mg}}{10 \text{ kg}}$$

   $$(2) \ 10 = 1x$$

   $$\frac{20}{1} = \frac{1x}{1}$$

   $$x = 20 \text{ mg}$$

3. $$\frac{20 \text{ mg}}{x \text{ cc}} = \frac{10 \text{ mg}}{0.5 \text{ cc}}$$

   $$10x = (0.5) \ 20$$

   $$\frac{10x}{10} = \frac{10}{10}$$

   $$x = 1 \text{ cc}$$

PRACTICE DOSAGE CALCULATION EXAMS

This is the format of the dosage calculation exams.

Each practice exam should be completed in one hour.

PRACTICE EXAM #1

Criteria for Grading Dosage Calculation Exams

1. Each problem must be set up in the fractional format.

2. Must show fractional format for each step in multiple step problems.

3. Must show units in formulas.

4. Must solve for x in each formula.

5. Always convert from one unit of measure to another by the shortest number of steps.

1. Ordered: 40 units
    Available: 100 units/ml
    How many <u>ml's</u> should be given? _____

2. Ordered: 3 mg
    Available: 1.5 mg/tablet
    How many <u>tablets</u> should be given? _____

3. Ordered: 1ss g̅r̅

    Available: s̅s̅ gr/tablet
    How many <u>tablets</u> should be given? _____

4. Ordered: 1000 mg
   Available: 250 mg/tablet
   How many <u>tablets</u> should be given? _____

5. Ordered: 5 mg
   Available: 10 mg/2 cc
   How many <u>cc's</u> should be given? _____

6. Ordered: 0.125 mg
   Available: 0.25 mg/tablet
   How many <u>tablets</u> should be given?

7. Ordered: 1/200 gr
   Available: 1/100 gr/tablet
   How many <u>tablets</u> should be given? _____

8. Ordered: 0.5 mg
   Available: 2 mg/ml
   How many <u>ml's</u> should be given? _____

9. Ordered: 0.3 gm
    Available: 300 mg/tablet
    How many <u>tablets</u> should be given? _____

10. Ordered: 150 mg
    Available: 1 gr/tablet
    How many <u>tablets</u> should be given? _____

11. Ordered: 30 mg
    Available: 6 mg/2 drams
    How many <u>cc's</u> should be given? _____

12. Ordered: 2 gr
    Available: 60 mg/tablet
    How many <u>tablets</u> should be given? _____

13. Ordered: 0.75 gm
    Available: 250 mg/tablet
    How many <u>tablets</u> should be given? _____

14. Ordered: 240 mg
    Available: 60 mg/cc
    How many <u>drams</u> should be given? _____

15. Ordered: 0.25 Gm
    Available: 125 mg/cc
    How many <u>cc's</u> should be given? _____

16. Ordered: 250 mg
    Available: 0.5 gm/tablet
    How many <u>tablets</u> should be given? _____

17. Ordered: 1/6 gr
    Available: 5 mg/cc
    How many <u>cc's</u> should be given? _____

18. Ordered: Two tablespoons of a liquid every 2 hours for 12 hours.
    How many <u>cc's</u> of the drug will the client receive over the 12 hour period? _____

19. A client weighing 110 lbs. is to receive a drug at the dosage of 2.5 mg/kg of body

weight. How many <u>mg</u> of the drug will the client receive? _____

20. A client is to receive 0.2 cc/kg of a drug every 2 hours. The client weighs 110 lbs.
How many <u>cc's</u> of drug will the client receive in 24 hours? _____

ANSWERS: Page 62

PRACTICE EXAM #2

Criteria for Grading Dosage Calculation Exams

1. Each problem must be set up in the fractional format.

2. Must show fractional format for each step in multiple step problems.

3. Must show units in formulas.

4. Must solve for x in each formula.

5. Always convert from one unit of measure to another by the shortest number of steps.

1. Ordered: 800,000 units
    Available: 2,000,000 units/10 cc
    How many cc's should be given? _____

2. Ordered: 60 mg
    Available: 30 mg/5 ml
    How many cc's should be given? _____

3. Ordered: 2 mg
    Available: 10 mg/2 cc
    How many cc's should be given? _____

4. Ordered: 2.5 gm
    Available: 1 gm/tab
    How many tablets should be given? _____

5. Ordered: 80 mg
    Available: 60 mg/0.6 ml
    How many cc's should be given? _____

6. Ordered: 0.25 mg
    Available: 0.05 mg/cc
    How many cc's will the client receive? _____

7. Ordered: XV gr
    Available: VIIss gr/tablet
    How many tablets should be given? _____

8. Ordered: 1/4 gr
    Available: 1/2 gr/tablet
    How many tablets should be given? _____

9. Ordered: gr 1/4
    Available: 30 mg/tab
    How many tablets should be given? _____

10. Ordered: 60 mg
    Available: 240 mg/dram
    How many cc's should be given? _____

11. Ordered: gr X
    Available: 300 mg tab
    How many tablets should be given? _____

12. Ordered: 15 meq
    Available: 5 meq/8 cc
    How many drams should be given? _____

13. Ordered: 0.5 gm
    Available: 250 mg/tab
    How many tablets should be given? _____

14. Ordered: 60 mg
    Available: 1/2 gr/tablet
    How many tablets should be given? _____

15. Ordered: 0.6 gm
    Available: 300 mg/cc
    How many cc's should be given? _____

16. Ordered: 15 meq
    Available: 5 meq/10 cc
    How many teaspoons should be given? _____

17. Ordered: 1 gm
    Available: 800 mg/2 cc
    How many <u>cc's</u> should be given? _____

18. A client receives 30 cc of a drug every 4 hours for 24 hours. How many drams will the client receive in 24 hrs? _____

19. A 66 lb. child is to receive a drug 2.5 mg/kg body weight. How many mg's will the child receive? _____

20. A sixty-six pound child is to receive 0.4 meq/kg of a drug. The drug is available in 2 meq/4 cc. How many cc's will be given? _____

ANSWERS: Page 66

PART E
PEDIATRIC MEDICATIONS

Steps:

1. Convert pounds to kilograms.

2. If weight is in ounces, convert ounces to nearest hundredth of a pound and add this to total pounds.

3. Since 16 oz. = 1 lb., change oz. to part of a pound by dividing by 16. Carry arithmetic out to three places and round off.

4. Then, convert total pounds to kilograms to nearest hundredths.

Example I:

O: Lasix 15 mg. po BID
A: 2 mg/kg

The infant weighs 16 lbs. 10 oz. How many mg will you give? Single dose? Bid?

$$\frac{.625}{10\ oz = 16|10.000}$$ = 0.63 lb. Child's wt. is 16.63 lbs.

```
10 oz = 16|10.000
16 oz.      96
            40
            32
            80
            80
             0
```

1. $\frac{1\ kg}{2.2\ lb.} = \frac{x\ kg}{16.63\ lb.}$

```
                                    7.559
2.2 x = 16.6      2.2|16.620   22|166.300
                               154
                               123
x = 7.559 kg    x = 7.56 kg    110
                               130
                               110
                               200
                               198
                                 2
```

2. $\frac{2\ mg}{1\ kg} = \frac{x\ mg}{7.56\ kg}$ BID 15.1 x 2 = 30.2 mg/day

x = 15.12 mg. single dose

Example II:

O: 115 mg/ml tid
A: 30 mg/kg/day in divided doses

Infant weighs 25 lbs. 4 oz. How many mg will nurse give in 1 day?

$\dfrac{4 \text{ oz.}}{16 \text{ oz.}}$ = $\dfrac{1}{4}$ or 0.25 = 0.3   Infant weighs 25.3 lbs.

1. $\dfrac{25.3 \text{ lb.}}{x \text{ kg}}$ = $\dfrac{2.2 \text{ lbs.}}{1 \text{ kg}}$

    2.2x = 25.3

    x = 11.5 kg

$$2.2\overline{)25.30}$$

$$\begin{array}{r} 11.5 \\ 22\,\overline{)2530} \\ \underline{22} \\ 33 \\ \underline{22} \\ 110 \\ \underline{110} \\ 0 \end{array}$$

2. $\dfrac{30 \text{ mg}}{1 \text{ kg}}$ = $\dfrac{x \text{ mg}}{11.5 \text{ kg}}$

    x = 30 x 11.5

    x = 345 mg

$$\begin{array}{r} 11.5 \\ \times\ 30 \\ \hline 345.0 \end{array}$$

1. A 20 pound, 8 ounce child is to receive Cosmegen 20 mcg/kg of body weight. How many micrograms should the child receive?

2. Ordered: Phenergan 1 mg/kg of body weight. How many mgs should you give to a 45 pound post-op child?

3. Ordered: 30 meq per kg. Client weighs 8 lb. 8 oz. How many meq should you give?

4. Ordered: 40 mg per kg of body wt.
    Available: 100 mg per 1cc
    How many cc's should you give to a 8 lb. 4 oz infant?

5. Ordered: 40 meq per kg of body wt. Your client weighs 8 lbs. 6 oz. How many meq should you give?

ANSWERS: Page 67

PART F
PARENTERAL MEDICATIONS

Directions for Calculating IV Flow Rates

A. To find flow rate stated in cc's per hour (if not given in the order):

$$\frac{\text{Total volume of solution in cc's}}{\text{Total number of hours to run}} = \frac{x \text{ cc's}}{\# \text{ hours}}$$

Example: 1000 cc IV solution ordered to infuse over 8 hours.

$$\frac{1000 \text{ cc}}{8 \text{ hrs.}} = 125$$

Answer: 125 cc/hour

This number (cc/hr) is used to calculate drops per minute.

*When answer does not come out evenly, round off to the nearest whole number. If 5 & greater round up. Below 5, round down.

Example: 1000 cc solution to infuse over 6 hours.

$$\frac{1000 \text{ cc}}{6 \text{ hrs.}} = 166.6 = 167$$

Answer: 167 cc or ml/hr

B. To find flow rate stated in drops per minute:

Drop factor is the number of drops it takes to equal 1 cc with a specific type of IV tubing. The drop factor is stated on the tubing package.

$$\frac{\text{cc/hr. x drop factor}}{60 \text{ min/hr}} = \text{gtts/min}$$

60 minutes/hr is a constant in this formula

Example: The drop factor is a 15 gtts/cc and the flow rate is 120cc/hr.

$$\frac{120\text{cc/hr x 15 gtts/cc}}{60 \text{ mins/hr}} = \frac{1800}{60} = 30 \text{ gtts/min}$$

Example: The drop factor is 20 gtts/cc and the flow rate is 100 cc/hr.

$$\frac{100\text{cc/hr} \times 20 \text{ gtts/cc}}{60 \text{ mins/hr}} = \frac{2000}{60} = 33 \text{ gtts/min}$$

*Remember, when answer does not come out even, round off to nearest whole number.

<u>Example:</u> 32.5 gtts = 33 gtts
       32.4 gtts = 32 gtts

IV Formulas

A. Amount of fluid per hour: ml/hr or cc/hr

$$\frac{\text{Total Volume}}{\text{Total \# of hrs. to infuse}} = \frac{TV}{TT} \qquad \text{Example:} \quad \frac{1000\text{cc}}{10\text{hr}} = 100\text{cc/hr}$$

B. How many drops per minute: gtts/min.

$$\frac{\text{ml/hr x drop factor (always given)}}{60 \text{ min/hr}}$$

Example: $\dfrac{100\text{cc} \times 20}{60} = \dfrac{2000}{60} = 33 \text{ gtts/min}$

C. How much drug in 1 ml (or cc) of fluid?

$$\frac{\text{Total amount of drug}}{\text{Total amount of fluid}} = \frac{TD}{TV}$$

Example: $\dfrac{500 \text{ mg of Keflin}}{1000 \text{ cc}} = 0.5 \text{ mg per cc}$

D. How much drug in hour?

1. $\dfrac{TV}{\#\text{cc/hr}} = TT$ (total time) Example: $\dfrac{1000 \text{ cc}}{100 \text{ cc/hr}} = 10 \text{ hr}$

2. $\dfrac{\text{Total amount of drug}}{\text{Total time (TT)}} = \dfrac{TD}{TT}$

    Example: $\dfrac{500 \text{ mg of Keflin}}{10 \text{ hr}} = 50 \text{ mg/hr}$

E.   What time of day will the IV end?

Current time + $\dfrac{TV}{ml/hr}$ = end time

Example: 9 AM + $\dfrac{1000 \text{ cc}}{100 \text{ cc/hr}}$ (10 hr)= 7 PM   9 AM + 10 = 7 PM, end time

With IV fluids - round off to the nearest whole number. With 5 or greater round up, less than 5 round down.

Example: 166.6 = 167 cc/hr
                163.4 = 163 cc/hr

Examples of Problems

1.   Ordered: 5 mg
     Available: 2 mg/ml
     How many ml do you give?

$\dfrac{2 \text{ mg}}{1 \text{ ml}} = \dfrac{5 \text{ mg}}{X \text{ ml}}$ 2X = 5   X = **2.5 ml**

2.   Ordered: 5 cc
     Available: 10 mg/cc

$\dfrac{10 \text{ mg}}{1 \text{ cc}} = \dfrac{X \text{ mg}}{5 \text{ cc}}$ 1X = 50   X = 50 mg

3.   IV Order: D_5W with 20 meq Kcl per liter to infuse at 50 cc/hour.

To prepare this solution, the nurse uses the stock preparation of Kcl (10 meq/5 cc) to add to the liter of D_5W to make the concentration ordered.

$\dfrac{10 \text{ meq}}{5 \text{ cc}} = \dfrac{20 \text{ meq}}{X \text{ cc}}$ 10 X = 100
                        X = **10 cc**

The drop factor is 60 gtts/cc. How many gtts/min will IV run?

$\dfrac{50 \text{ cc/hr} \times 60 \text{ (drop factor)}}{60 \text{ min.}}$

How much fluid will client receive in 24 hours?

$\dfrac{50 \text{ cc}}{1 \text{ hr.}}$ x 24 hours = 1200 cc

How many meq of Kcl will client receive in one hour?

$\dfrac{20 \text{ meq}}{1000 \text{ cc}}$ = $\dfrac{X \text{ meq}}{50 \text{ cc}}$ (amount of solution received in one hour)

1000 X = 1000

X = **1 meq**

4. Ordered: 2 mg/kg
   Client weighed: 44 lbs.
   How many mg will client receive?

   $$\frac{2.2 \text{ lbs}}{1 \text{ kg}} = \frac{44 \text{ lbs}}{X \text{ kg}}$$

   $$2.2 X = 44$$
   $$X = 20 \text{ kg}$$

   $$\frac{2 \text{ mg}}{1 \text{ kg}} = \frac{X \text{ mg}}{20 \text{ kg}}$$

   $$X = \textbf{40 mg}$$

5. Ordered: $D_5 1/2NS$ to infuse 2 liters over 16 hours. How many cc's/hr will be infused per hour?

   $$\frac{2000 \text{ cc}}{16 \text{ hrs.}} = \textbf{125 cc/hr}$$

PRACTICE EXAM #4

Dosage Calculation Directions:

1.   At the end of each step round the answer to the nearest hundredths before proceeding to the next step.
2.   If the final answer is less than one, the answer should be rounded off to hundredths, Example .6666   .67
3.   If the final answer is greater than one, the answer should be rounded to tenths, Example 1.812   1.8
4.   In IV problems, round to the nearest whole number. Therefore, you must round the final answer up if equal to or greater than .5 and round down if less than .5. See example, page 46. If the question states that the IV solution is administered by IV pump, the final answer must be rounded to the nearest hundredth.

5.   **ALL WORK MUST BE SHOWN!**

6.   The answer must be clearly identified by <u>placing answer on the blank line</u> or circled on the worksheet by the question.

1.   Order: IV of $D_5$1/2NS at 100 cc/hr (20 gtts/cc)
     How many drops per minute? _____

2.   Order: 500 cc of LR with 20 meq Kcl over 8 hours (15 gtts/cc)
     How many drops per minute? _____

3.   Order: 1.5 Gm po
     Available: 500 mg/tablet
     How many tablets will you give? _____

4.   Order: gr 1/6 IM
     Available: 30 mg/cc
     How many cc's will you give? _____

5. Order: 0.5 gm po
   Available: 250 mg/cc
   How many cc's will you give? _____

6. Order: 200,000 u IM
   Available: 500,000 u/5 cc
   How many cc's will you give? _____

7. Order: 200 mg IM
   Available: 500 mg/cc
   How many cc's will you give? _____

8. Order: 750 mcg po
   Available: 0.5 mg/tablet
   How many tablets will you give? _____

9. Order: 4 mg IM
   Available: gr 1/20/cc
   How many cc's will you give? _____

10. Order: 250 mcg IM
    Available: 1 mg per 2 cc
    How many cc's do you give? _____

ANSWERS: Page 70

PRACTICE EXAM #5

<u>Dosage Calculation Directions:</u>

1.   At the end of each step round the answer to the nearest hundredths before
        proceeding to the next step.
2.   If the final answer is less than one, the answer should be rounded off to
        hundredths, Example .6<u>6</u>66   .67
3.   If the final answer is greater than one, the answer should be rounded to
        tenths, Example 1.<u>8</u>12   1.8
4.   In IV problems, round to the nearest whole number. Therefore, you must
        round the final answer <u>up</u> if equal to or greater than .5 and round <u>down</u> if
        less than .5. See example, page 46. If the question states that the IV
        solution is administered by IV pump, the final answer must be rounded to
        the nearest hundredth.

5.   **ALL WORK MUST BE SHOWN!**

6.   The answer must be clearly identified by <u>placing answer on the blank line</u> or
        circled on the worksheet by the question.

Order: 1000 cc of D$_5$W to infuse over 12 hours (20 gtts/cc)
         1.   How many cc per hour? _____
         2.   How many drops per minute? _____

Order: 1000 cc of D$_5$NS to infuse at 125 cc/hr (60 gtts/cc)
         3.   How many drops per minute? _____

Order: 100 cc D$_5$W with 2 gm Keflin to infuse in 1 hour (15 gtts/cc)
         4.   How many drops per minute? _____
         5.   How many mg of Keflin in 1 cc? _____

Order: 500 cc LR to infuse over 10 hours (60 gtts/cc)
         6.   How many cc per hour? _____
         7.   How many drops per minute? _____

Order: 500 cc D$_5$W with 500 mg Aminophyllin to infuse at 150 cc/hr (20 gtts/cc).
   8.   How many drops per minute? _____

Order: 1000 cc LR to infuse over 10 hours (60 gtts/cc)
   9.   How many cc per hour? _____
   10.   How many drops per minute? _____

Order: 250 cc NS to infuse at 50 cc/hour - started at 9 a.m. (60 gtts/cc)
   11.   How many drops per minute? _____
   12.   At what time of day will the NS have infused? _____

13.   Order: gr ½ IM
      Available: 15 mg/ml
      How many ml's will you give? _____

14.   Order: 2 gm po
      Available: 500 mg/tablet
      How many tablets will you give? _____

15.   Order: 4000u sq
      Available: 5000u/0.5 ml
      How many ml's will you give? _____

16.   Order: 10 mg po
      Available: 5 mg/dram
      How many ml's will you give? _____

17. Order: gr 1/4 IM
     Available: gr 1/6 per ml
     How many ml's will you give? _____

18. Order: 250 mcg
     Available: 0.25 mg/tablet
     How many tablets will you give? _____

19. Order: gr 1ss IM
     Available: 50 mg/ml
     How many ml's will you give? _____

20. Order: 30 mg/kg po (Client weighs 110 lbs.)
     Available: 500 mg/capsule
     How many capsule(s) will you give? _____

ANSWERS: Page 70

PRACTICE EXAM #6

Dosage Calculation Directions:

1. At the end of each step round the answer to the nearest hundredths before proceeding to the next step.
2. If the final answer is less than one, the answer should be rounded off to hundredths, Example .6666   .67
3. If the final answer is greater than one, the answer should be rounded to tenths, Example 1.812   1.8
4. In IV problems, round to the nearest whole number. Therefore, you must round the final answer <u>up</u> if equal to or greater than .5 and round <u>down</u> if less than .5. See example, page 46. If the question states that the IV solution is administered by IV pump, the final answer must be rounded to the nearest hundredth.

5. **ALL WORK MUST BE SHOWN!**

6. The answer must be clearly identified by <u>placing answer on the blank line</u> or circled on the worksheet by the question.

1. Order: IV of D5W to infuse at 140 cc/hr (20 gtts/cc)
    How many drops per minute?

2. Order: 1000 cc of D$_5$LR with 20 u Pitocin over 10 hours (15 gtts/cc)
    How many drops per minute? _____

3. Order: gr 1/8 IM
    Available: 15 mg/ml
    How many ml's will you give? _____

4. Order: 1 gm po
    Available: 250 mg/tablet
    How many tablet(s) will you give? _____

5. Order: 3000 u sq
    Available: 5000 u/0.5 ml
    How many ml's will you give? _____

6.   Order: 15 mg po
     Available: 5 mg/dram
     How many ml's will you give? _____

7.   Order: gr 1/6 IM
     Available: gr 1/4 per 2 ml
     How many ml's will you give? _____

8.   Order: 750 mcg po
     Available: 0.25 mg/tablet
     How many tablet(s) will you give? _____

9.   Order: 3 gr IM
     Available: 90 mg/ml
     How many ml's will you give? _____

10. Order: 7 mg/kg (Client weighs 11 lbs.)
     Available: 70 mg/ml
     How many ml's will you give? _____

11. Order: IV of NS to infuse at 90 cc/hr (12 gtts/cc)
     How many drops per minute? _____

12. Order: 1000 c of LR to infuse over 5 hours (20 gtts/cc)
     How many drops per minute? _____

13.   Order: gr 1/4 IM
      Available: 10 mg/ml
      How many ml's will you give? _____

14.   Order: 1.5 gm po
      Available: 750 mg/tablet
      How many tablet(s) will you give? _____

15.   Order: 5000 u sq
      Available: 10,000 u/ml
      How many ml's will you give? _____

16.   Order: 7.5 mg po
      Available: 5 mg/dram
      How many ml's will you give? _____

17.   Order: gr 1/150 IM
      Available: gr 1/200 per ml
      How many ml's will you give? _____

18.   Order: 125 mcg po
      Available: 0.25 mg/tablet
      How many tablet(s) will you give? _____

19. Order: gr 1ss IM
    Available: 60 mg/ml
    How many ml's will you give? _____

20. Order: 15 mg/kg IM (Client weighs 154 lbs.)
    Available: 500 mg/ml
    How many ml's will you give? _____

ANSWERS: Page 70

Answers to Basic Math

Roman Numerals #1

1.	16	6.	1120
2.	412	7.	LIV
3.	47	8.	XXIX
4.	21	9.	LXXXIII
5.	44	10.	$\overline{\text{iiss}}$

Fractions #2

1. $7\frac{1}{2}$

2. $2\frac{1}{6}$

3. $1\frac{3}{4}$

4. $3\frac{2}{3}$

5. $1\frac{7}{8}$

6. $7\frac{2}{5}$

7. $\frac{2}{3}$

8. $\frac{1}{3}$

9. $\frac{1}{4}$

10. $1\frac{49}{80}$

11. $\frac{43}{45}$

12. $1\frac{3}{7}$

13. $\frac{1}{6}$

14. 0

15. $\frac{4}{21}$

16. $\frac{7}{12}$

17. $1\frac{1}{8}$

18. $\frac{3}{625}$

19. $\frac{1}{2}$

20. 5

21. 15

22. $\frac{4}{9}$

Decimals #3

1. 0.75	11. 2.64	23. 0.04
2. 0.5	12. 1.84	24. 32
3. 0.375	13. 0.63	25. 0.45
4. 0.6<u>7</u>	14. 0.01	26. 0.01
5. $\frac{54}{100} = \frac{27}{50}$	15. 2.42	27. 9.9
	16. 0.43	28. 50.1
6. $\frac{154}{1000} = \frac{77}{500}$	17. 0.3749	29. 5620
7. $\frac{60}{100} = \frac{3}{5}$	18. 0.00369	30. 79
	19. 2.3635	
8. $\frac{2}{10} = \frac{1}{5}$	20. 0.006	
9. 2.24	21. 0.8	
10. 1.02	22. 0.62	

Metric Systems #4	Household System #5
1. 7000 gm 2. 50 ml 3. 2,500 mg 4. 5,070 gm 5. 0.0005 liter 6. 19.3 ml. 7. 1,340,000 mg 8. 0.0037 gm	1. 120 gtts 2. 4.5 t or $4\frac{1}{2}$ t 3. $\frac{3}{4}$ or 0.75 t 4. $2\frac{1}{2}$ or 2.5 oz. 5. 16 T $\quad \dfrac{8\ oz.}{x\ T} = \dfrac{1\ oz.}{2\ T}$ $\qquad x = 16\ T$ 6. 4 T $\quad \dfrac{12\ t}{x\ T} = \dfrac{3\ t}{1\ T}$ $\qquad \dfrac{3x}{3} = \dfrac{12}{3} = 4\ T$

Practice Exam #1 Answers

1. $\quad \dfrac{100\ units}{1\ ml} = \dfrac{40\ units}{x\ ml}$ $\quad 100\ x = 40$ $\quad \dfrac{100x}{100} = \dfrac{40}{100}$ $\quad x = 0.4\ ml$	2. $\quad \dfrac{1.5\ mg}{1\ tablet} = \dfrac{3\ mg}{x\ tablets}$ $\quad 1.5x = 3$ $\quad \dfrac{1.5x}{1.5} = \dfrac{3}{1.5}$ $\quad x = 2\ tablets$
3. $\dfrac{\frac{1}{2}\ gr}{1\ tab} = \dfrac{1\frac{1}{2}\ gr}{x\ tab}$ $\frac{1}{2}\ x = 1\frac{1}{2}\ x$ $\dfrac{\frac{1}{2}\ x}{\frac{1}{2}} = \dfrac{1\frac{1}{2}\ x}{\frac{1}{2}}$ $x = 3\ tablets$	4. $\dfrac{250\ mg}{1\ tablet} = \dfrac{1000\ mg}{x\ tablet}$ $250x = 1000$ $\dfrac{250x}{250} = \dfrac{1000}{250}$ $x = 4\ tablets$

5.	6.
$\dfrac{10\ mg}{2\ cc} = \dfrac{5\ mg}{x\ cc}$	$\dfrac{0.25\ mg}{1\ tablet} = \dfrac{0.125\ mg}{x\ tablet}$
$10x = 10$	$0.25x = 0.125$
$\dfrac{10x}{10} = \dfrac{10}{10}$	$\dfrac{0.25x}{0.25} = \dfrac{0.125}{0.25}$
$x = 1\ cc$	$x = 0.5\ tablet$
7.	8.
$\dfrac{1/100\ gr}{1\ tablet} = \dfrac{1/200\ gr}{x\ tablet}$	$\dfrac{2\ mg}{1\ ml} = \dfrac{0.5\ mg}{x\ ml}$
$1/100\ x = 1/200$	$2x = 0.5$
$\dfrac{1/100x}{1/100} = \dfrac{1/200}{1/100}$	$\dfrac{2x}{2} = \dfrac{0.5}{2}$
$x = \dfrac{1}{2}\ tablet$	$x = 0.25\ ml$
9.	
$\dfrac{300\ mg}{1\ tablet} = \dfrac{0.3\ gm}{x\ tablet}$	
A. $\dfrac{1000\ mg}{1\ gm} = \dfrac{x\ mg}{0.3\ gm}$	B. $\dfrac{300\ mg}{1\ tablet} = \dfrac{300\ mg}{1\ tablet}$
$x = 0.3 \times 1000$	$300x = 300$
$x = 300\ mg$	$\dfrac{300x}{300} = \dfrac{300}{300}$
	$x = 1\ tablet$
10.	
$\dfrac{1\ gr}{1\ tablet} = \dfrac{150\ mg}{x\ tablet}$	
A. $\dfrac{60\ mg}{1\ gr} = \dfrac{150\ mg}{x\ gr}$	B. $\dfrac{1\ gr}{1\ tablet} = \dfrac{2.5\ gr}{x\ tablet}$
$60x = 150$	$x = 2.5\ tablets$
$\dfrac{60x}{60} = \dfrac{150}{60}$	
$x = 2.5\ gr$	

11. $\dfrac{6 \text{ mg}}{2 \text{ drams}} = \dfrac{30 \text{ mg}}{x \text{ cc}}$	
A. $\dfrac{1 \text{ dram}}{4 \text{ cc}} = \dfrac{2 \text{ drams}}{x \text{ cc}}$ $x = 8 \text{ cc}$	B. $\dfrac{6 \text{ mg}}{8 \text{ cc}} = \dfrac{30 \text{ mg}}{x \text{ cc}}$ $6x = 30 \times 8$ $6x = 240$ $x = 40 \text{ cc}$
12. $\dfrac{60 \text{ mg}}{1 \text{ tablet}} = \dfrac{2 \text{ gr}}{x \text{ tablet}}$	
A. $\dfrac{1 \text{ gr}}{60 \text{ mg}} = \dfrac{2 \text{ gr}}{x \text{ mg}}$ $x = 2 \times 60$ $x = 120 \text{ mg}$	B. $\dfrac{60 \text{ mg}}{1 \text{ tablet}} = \dfrac{120 \text{ mg}}{x \text{ tablet}}$ $60x = 120$ $\dfrac{60x}{60} = \dfrac{120}{60}$ $x = 2 \text{ tablets}$
13. $\dfrac{250 \text{ mg}}{1 \text{ tablet}} = \dfrac{0.75 \text{ gm}}{x \text{ tablet}}$	
A. $\dfrac{1000 \text{ mg}}{1 \text{ gm}} = \dfrac{x \text{ mg}}{0.75 \text{ gm}}$ $x = 0.75 \text{ gm}$ $x = 0.75 \times 1000$ $x = 750 \text{ mg}$	B. $\dfrac{250 \text{ mg}}{1 \text{ tablet}} = \dfrac{750 \text{ mg}}{x \text{ tablet}}$ $250x = 750$ $x = 3 \text{ tablets}$
14. $\dfrac{60 \text{ mg}}{1 \text{ cc}} = \dfrac{240 \text{ mg}}{x \text{ dram}}$	
A. $\dfrac{1 \text{ dram}}{4 \text{ cc}} = \dfrac{x \text{ dram}}{1 \text{ cc}}$ $4x = 1$ $\dfrac{4x}{4} = \dfrac{1}{4}$ $x = 0.25 \text{ dram}$	B. $\dfrac{60 \text{ mg}}{0.25 \text{ dram}} = \dfrac{240 \text{ mg}}{x \text{ dram}}$ $60x = 60$ $\dfrac{60x}{60} = \dfrac{60}{60}$ $x = 1 \text{ dram}$

15. $\dfrac{125 \text{ mg}}{1 \text{ cc}} = \dfrac{0.25 \text{ gm}}{\text{x cc}}$	
A. $\dfrac{1000 \text{ mg}}{1 \text{ gm}} = \dfrac{\text{x mg}}{0.25 \text{ gm}}$ x = .25 x 1000 x = 250 mg	B. $\dfrac{125 \text{ mg}}{1 \text{ cc}} = \dfrac{250 \text{ mg}}{\text{x cc}}$ 125x = 250 $\dfrac{125x}{125} = \dfrac{250}{125}$ x = 2 cc
16. $\dfrac{0.5 \text{ gm}}{1 \text{ tablet}} = \dfrac{250 \text{ mg}}{\text{x tablet}}$	
A. $\dfrac{1000 \text{ mg}}{1 \text{ gm}} = \dfrac{250 \text{ mg}}{\text{x gm}}$ 1000x = 250 $\dfrac{1000x}{1000} = \dfrac{250}{1000}$ x = 0.25 gm	B. $\dfrac{0.5 \text{ gm}}{1 \text{ tablet}} = \dfrac{0.25 \text{ gm}}{\text{x tablet}}$ 0.5x = 0.25 $\dfrac{0.5x}{0.5} = \dfrac{0.25}{0.5}$ x = 0.5 tablet
17. $\dfrac{5 \text{ mg}}{1 \text{ cc}} = \dfrac{1/6 \text{ gr}}{\text{x cc}}$	
A. $\dfrac{60 \text{ mg}}{1 \text{ gr}} = \dfrac{\text{x mg}}{1/6 \text{ gr}}$ x = 1/6 x 60 x = 10 mg	B. $\dfrac{5 \text{ mg}}{1 \text{ cc}} = \dfrac{10 \text{ mg}}{\text{x cc}}$ 5x = 10 $\dfrac{5x}{5} = \dfrac{10}{5}$ x = 2 cc
18. $\dfrac{2 \text{ Tbsp}}{2 \text{ hr}} = \dfrac{\text{x cc}}{12 \text{ hr}}$	
A. $\dfrac{1 \text{ Tbsp}}{15 \text{ cc}} = \dfrac{2 \text{ Tbsp}}{\text{x cc}}$ x = 15 x 2 x = 30 cc	B. $\dfrac{30 \text{ cc}}{2 \text{ hr}} = \dfrac{\text{x cc}}{12 \text{ hr}}$ 2x = 360 $\dfrac{2x}{2} = \dfrac{360}{2}$ x = 180 cc

19. $\dfrac{2.5 \text{ mg}}{1 \text{ Kg}} = \dfrac{\text{x mg}}{110 \text{ lb}}$	
A. $\dfrac{2.2 \text{ lb}}{1 \text{ Kg}} = \dfrac{110 \text{ lb}}{\text{x Kg}}$ 2.2x = 110 $\dfrac{2.2\text{x}}{2.2} = \dfrac{110}{2.2}$ x = 50 Kg	B. $\dfrac{2.5 \text{ mg}}{1 \text{ Kg}} = \dfrac{\text{x mg}}{50 \text{ Kg}}$ x = 50 x 2.5 x = 125 mg
20. $\dfrac{0.2 \text{ cc}}{1 \text{ Kg}} = \dfrac{\text{x cc}}{110 \text{ lbs}}$	
A. $\dfrac{1 \text{ Kg}}{2.2 \text{ lbs}} = \dfrac{\text{x Kg}}{110 \text{ lbs}}$ 2.2x = 110 $\dfrac{2.2\text{x}}{2.2} = \dfrac{110}{2.2}$ x = 50 Kg	B. $\dfrac{0.2 \text{ cc}}{1 \text{ Kg}} = \dfrac{\text{x cc}}{50 \text{ Kg}}$ x = 0.2 x 50 x = 10 cc C. $\dfrac{10 \text{ cc}}{2 \text{ hr}} = \dfrac{\text{x cc}}{24 \text{ hr}}$ 2x = 10 x 24 $\dfrac{2\text{x}}{2} = \dfrac{240}{2}$ x = 120 cc q 24 hrs

Practice Exam #2 Answers

1.	4 cc	11.	2 tablets
2.	10 cc	12.	6 drams
3.	0.4 cc	13.	2 tablets
4.	2.5 tablets	14.	2 tablets
5.	0.8 cc	15.	2 cc
6.	5 cc	16.	6 teaspoons
7.	2 tablets	17.	2.5 cc
8.	0.5 tablet	18.	45 drams
9.	0.5 tablet	19.	75 mg
10.	1 cc	20.	24 cc's

These practice problems should assist the student to identify strengths and weaknesses in math skills. There are appropriate resources in the Learning Resource Center to assist with identified weakness. Refer to page 6 in this booklet.

Answers to Practice Exam #3 (Pediatric Problems)

1.   ① $\dfrac{8\ oz}{16\ oz} = .5$ ② $\dfrac{2.2\ lb}{1\ Kg.} = \dfrac{20.5\ lb}{x\ Kg}$ ③ $\dfrac{20\ meq}{1\ Kg} = \dfrac{x\ meq}{9.32\ Kg}$

                           x = 9.32 Kg   **x = 186.4**

---

2.   ① $\dfrac{2.2\ lb.}{1\ kg} = \dfrac{45\ lb.}{x\ kg}$

               $2.2x = 45$

          x = 20.45 kg

            $\dfrac{20.45}{2.2\ |\ 45.000} = 20.5$

                 $\underline{44}$
                 100
                   $\underline{88}$
                 120
                 $\underline{110}$
                 100

   ② $\dfrac{1\ mg}{1\ kg} = \dfrac{x\ mg}{20.45\ kg}$ $\dfrac{88}{12}$

   x = 20.45 = 20.5 mg of phenergan

---

3.   ① $\dfrac{1\ kg}{2.2\ lb.} = \dfrac{x\ kg}{8.5\ lb}$ $\dfrac{8\ oz}{16\ oz.} = \dfrac{1}{2} = 0.5$

             $2.2x = 8.5$ $\dfrac{3.863}{2.2\ |\ 8.500} = 3.86$

        x = 3.86 kg $\underline{66}$
                             190
                            $\underline{176}$
   ② $\dfrac{30\ meq}{1\ kg} = \dfrac{x\ meq}{3.86\ kg}$ 140
                             $\underline{132}$
                                 80

      $x = 30 \times 3.86$ $\underline{66}$
                            14

     x = 115.8 meq 3.86
                            $\underline{\times\ 30}$
                            115.8

4. ① $\dfrac{4\ oz}{16\ oz}$ = 0.25 = 0.3 $\dfrac{.25}{16\ |4.00}$ = 0.3

                                          $\underline{32}$

                                          80

                                          $\underline{80}$

     $\dfrac{1\ kg}{2.2\ lb}$ = $\dfrac{x\ kg}{8.3\ lb}$ $\dfrac{3.772}{2.2\ |8.300}$ = 3.77

                                          $\underline{66}$

     2.2x = 8.3   170

                                          $\underline{154}$

     x = 3.8 kg   160

                                          $\underline{154}$

                                          160

                                                  $\underline{88}$

                                                  72

  ② $\dfrac{40\ mg}{1\ kg}$ = $\dfrac{x\ mg}{3.77\ kg}$ 3.77

                                 $\underline{x\ \ 40}$

                                 150.8

     x = 40 x 3.77

     x = 150.8 mg

  ③ $\dfrac{100\ mg}{1\ cc}$ = $\dfrac{150.8\ mg}{x\ cc}$ $\dfrac{1.508}{100\ |150.800}$

                                          $\underline{100}$

     100x = 152   508

                                          $\underline{500}$

     x = 1.508 cc = 1.5 cc   800

                                                  $\underline{800}$

                                                  0

5.　① $\frac{1 \text{ kg}}{2.2 \text{ lb}} = \frac{x \text{ kg}}{8.4 \text{ lb}}$　$\frac{6 \text{ oz.}}{16 \text{ oz.}} = 0.375$

$2.2x = 8.4$

x = 3.82kg

$\frac{.375}{16|6.000} = 0.4$
$\underline{48}$
1200
$\underline{112}$
80
$\underline{80}$

$\frac{3.828}{2.2|8.40} = 3.82$
$\underline{66}$
1800
$\underline{176}$
40
$\underline{22}$
180
$\underline{176}$
4

② $\frac{40 \text{ meq}}{1 \text{ kg}} = \frac{x \text{ meq}}{3.82 \text{ kg}}$

3.8
$\underline{\times 40}$
152.0

$x = 40 \times 3.82$

x = 152.8 meq

Answers to Practice Exam #4 (IV Problems)

1. 33 gtts/minute

2. 16 gtts/minute

3. 3 Tabs

4. .33 cc

5. 2 cc

6. 2 cc

7. 0.4 cc

8. 1.5 tablets

9. 1.3 cc

10. 0.5 cc

Answers to Practice Exam #5		**Answers to Practice Exam #6**	
1.	83 cc/hr	1.	47 gtts/minute
2.	28 gtts/minute	2.	25 gtts/minute
3.	125 gtts/minute	3.	0.5 ml
4.	25 gtts/minute	4.	4 tablets
5.	20 mg	5.	0.3 ml
6.	50 cc/hour	6.	12 ml
7.	50 gtts/minute	7.	1.3 ml
8.	50 gtts/minute	8.	3 tablets
9.	100 cc/hour	9.	2 ml
10.	100 gtts/minute	10.	0.5 ml
11.	50 gtts/minute	11.	18 gtts/minute
12.	2 p.m.	12.	67 gtts/minute
13.	2 ml	13.	1.5 ml
14.	4 tablets	14.	2 tablets
15.	0.4 ml	15.	0.5 ml
16.	8 ml	16.	6 ml
17.	1.5 ml	17.	1.3 ml
18.	1 tablet	18.	0.5 tablets
19.	1.8 ml	19.	1.5 ml
20.	3 capsules	20.	2.1 ml

Part G IV DRIP CALCULATIONS

Calculation of Weight Based IV Drips

Drugs can be administered to clients in continuous IV drips. The medication bag/syringe is labeled with the concentration of medication in the solution (i.e. units/ml, mcg/ml, meq/ml). The medication order will be used to determine the setup of the problem. Ratio and proportions can be set up to solve these problems, and depending upon the complexity of the order several steps may be needed. The following examples will show you the basis for solving these problems.

A. When the order is written as mg/hr.

Example
Order: Fentanyl 5 mg/hr. The bag is labeled 250 mg in 500 ml of solution.
How fast will the IV need to be infused to give the correct dose?

1. The IV rate will be as an hourly rate, so no conversion needs to be made for time. If the order was written with a different time, you would need to calculate the mg/hr. (use ratio and proportion)

2. Put the problem in ratio and proportion.

$$\frac{5 \text{ mg}}{x \text{ ml}} = \frac{250 \text{ mg}}{500 \text{ ml}} \qquad 5 (500) = 250 \text{ x} \qquad \frac{2500}{250} \qquad x = 10 \text{ ml/hr} \quad \text{IV rate}$$

B. The order may be written as unit of measurement/ Kg of weight/ hour.

Example
Order: Heparin 100 units/Kg/hr. The label on the solution reads 10,000 units/50 ml. The patient weighs 70 Kg. How fast should the solution run to give the correct dosage?

1.   First you need the total dosage/hr.
Dose (units/hr) x weight in Kg equals the hourly dose. If the weight is in lbs, that must be converted to Kg first.

100 units x 70 Kg = 7,000 units/hr

2.   Now put the dose in ratio and proportion with the concentration.

$$\frac{7,000 \text{ units}}{x \text{ ml}} = \frac{10,000 \text{ units}}{50 \text{ ml}} \quad 10,000x = 50 (7,000) \quad x= \frac{350,000}{10,000} \quad x= 35 \text{ ml/hr} \quad \text{rate}$$

C. When the order is written as unit of measurement/Kg of wt/minute.

Example
Order: Dopamine 20 mcg/Kg/minute. The bag is labeled Dopamine 100 mg/50 ml. The patient weighs 88 lbs. How fast will the IV run to give the dose?

1.   First because the weight is in lbs, you must convert lbs. to Kg.
(88 lbs = 40 Kg)

2. Find the hourly dose.   Because it is written in mcg/K/min you must multiply by 60 minutes to get the hourly dose.

    20mcg x 40 Kg x 60 minutes = 48,000 mcg/hr

3. Note that the concentration is in mg/ml not mcg, so you must convert to obtain like units of measure.

    $\dfrac{100\ mg}{x\ mcg} = \dfrac{1mg}{1000\ mcg}$ $\qquad\qquad$ x=100,000 mcg/ml

4. Lastly set the problem up in ratio and proportion.

$\dfrac{100,000\ mcg}{50\ ml} = \dfrac{48,000\ mcg/hr}{x\ ml}$ $\quad$ 100,000x = 2,400,000 $\quad$ x = 24 ml / hr IV rate

Practice Exam #7

1. Order: Morphine 5 mg/hr. The syringe is labeled 100 mg/ 100 ml. How fast will the IV run to deliver the correct dosage? _____
2. Order: Heparin 50 units/Kg/hr. The solution is labeled 1000 units/ ml. The patient weighs 10 Kg. What is the correct rate? _____
3. Order: Dobutamine 10 mcg/Kg/min. The bag is labeled 1 mg/ ml. The patient weighs 23 Kg. What is the correct rate? _____
4. Order: Pitocin 5 miliunits/minute. The bag is labeled 10 units/liter. What is the correct rate?_____
5. Order: Ritodrine 10 miliunits/ Kg/ min. The bag is labeled 100 units/100 ml. The patient weighs 198 lbs. What is the correct rate?_____

ANSWERS: pg. 73

PRACTICE EXAM #7 ANSWERS

1. $\dfrac{5\ mg}{x\ ml} = \dfrac{100\ mg}{100\ ml}$

    $100x = 500\ ml$

    $x = \dfrac{500}{100} = 5\ ml/hr.\ rate$

2. a. 50 units x 10 Kg x 60 min = 30,000 units/hr

    b. $\dfrac{30,000\ units}{x\ ml} = \dfrac{1000\ units}{1\ ml}$

       $1000x = 30,000\ (1)$

       $x = \dfrac{30,000}{1000} = 30\ ml/hr\ IV\ rate$

3. a. 10 mcg x 23 kg x 60 min = 13,800 mcg/hr

    b. $\dfrac{13,800\ mcg}{x\ ml} = \dfrac{1\ mg}{1\ ml}$

       NOTE: You must have like units of 1mg = 1000 mcg

    c. $\dfrac{13,800\ mcg}{x\ ml} = \dfrac{1000\ mcg}{1\ ml}$

       $1000x = 13,800\ (1)$

       $x = \dfrac{13,800}{1000} = $ 13.8 ml/hr rate on an IV pump
       OR
       14 ml/hr rate if it is on a free flowing IV

4. a. 5 miliunits x 60 min = 300 mililunits/hr

    b. $\dfrac{300\ mu}{x\ ml} = \dfrac{10\ u}{1L}$ 10 units = 10,000 mu
    1 Liter = 1000 ml

       $\dfrac{300\ mu}{x\ ml} = \dfrac{10,000}{1,000}$

       $10,000x = 300,000$
       $x = \dfrac{300,000}{10,000}$

       $x = $ 30 ml rate

5.　　a.　198 lbs. = 90 Kg

　　　b.　10 mu x 90 K x 60 min = 54,000 mu/hr

$$\frac{54{,}000 \text{ mu}}{x \text{ ml}} = \frac{100 \text{ units}}{100 \text{ mL}} \qquad 100 \text{ units} = 100{,}000 \text{ mu}$$

$$\frac{54{,}000 \text{ mu}}{x \text{ ml}} = \frac{100{,}000 \text{ mu}}{100 \text{ mL}}$$

$$5{,}400{,}000 = 100{,}000x$$

$$\frac{5{,}400{,}000}{100{,}000} = x$$

x = 54 mL/hr rate

Printed in Great Britain
by Amazon

37137926R00044